P9-BIJ-657

DRUG
DANGERS

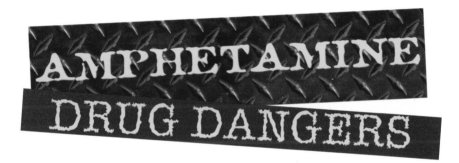

AMPHETAMINE
DRUG DANGERS

Michael J. Pellowski

Enslow Publishers, Inc.

40 Industrial Road   PO Box 38
Box 398   Aldershot
Berkeley Heights, NJ 07922   Hants GU12 6BP
USA   UK

http://www.enslow.com

J
362.29
c.1

Copyright © 2000 by Enslow Publishers, Inc.

All rights reserved.

No part of this book may be reproduced by any means
without the written permission of the publisher.

Library of Congress Cataloging-in-Publication Data

Pellowski, Michael.
    Amphetamine drug dangers / Michael J. Pellowski.
        p. cm. — (Drug dangers)
    Includes bibliographical references and index.
    Summary: Discusses amphetamines, their misuse, abuse, and dangers.
    ISBN 0-7660-1321-9
    1. Amphetamine abuse—United States Juvenile literature.
    2. Teenagers—Substance use—United States Juvenile literature.
    [1. Amphetamines. 2. Drug abuse.] I. Title. II. Series.
    HV5822.A5P45   2000
    362.29'9—dc21   99-36152
                                                              CIP

Printed in the United States of America

10 9 8 7 6 5 4 3 2 1

To our Readers:
All Internet addresses in this book were active and appropriate when we
went to press. Any comments or suggestions can be sent by e-mail to
Comments@enslow.com or to the address on the back cover.

Photo Credits: Copyright © 1998, Williams & Wilkins, A Waverly Company,
p, 40; Corel Corporation, pp. 9, 11, 20, 24, 38, 49; Díamar Interactive Corp.,
p. 34; National Archives, pp. 16, 22, 37, 41; Photofest, p. 6; Skjold
Photographs, pp. 43, 47.

Cover Photo: © Corel Corporation

contents

Titles in the **Drug Dangers** series:

Alcohol Drug Dangers
ISBN 0-7660-1159-3

Amphetamine Drug Dangers
ISBN 0-7660-1321-9

Crack and Cocaine Drug Dangers
ISBN 0-7660-1155-0

Diet Pill Drug Dangers
ISBN 0-7660-1158-5

Ecstasy and Other Designer Drug Dangers
ISBN 0-7660-1322-7

Herbal Drug Dangers
ISBN 0-7660-1319-7

Heroin Drug Dangers
ISBN 0-7660-1156-9

Inhalant Drug Dangers
ISBN 0-7660-1153-4

LSD, PCP, and Hallucinogen Drug Dangers
ISBN 0-7660-1318-9

Marijuana Drug Dangers
ISBN 0-7660-1214-X

Speed and Methamphetamine Drug Dangers
ISBN 0-7660-1157-7

Steroid Drug Dangers
ISBN 0-7660-1154-2

Tobacco and Nicotine Drug Dangers
ISBN 0-7660-1317-0

Tranquilizer, Barbiturate, and Downer
Drug Dangers
ISBN 0-7660-1320-0

one

Life in the Fast Lane

He was the undisputed king of rock and roll. He was and still is loved and adored by millions of rock music fans all over the world. He had talent, good looks, wealth, and fame. Some said he had it all. No person ever had more to live for than Elvis Presley—the King.

The Costly Price of Fame

Unfortunately, there was also a dark side to this multitalented performer's success. This superstar had problems with certain types of drugs, among them amphetamines. Drug use may have contributed heavily to the tragic and untimely death in August 1977 of Elvis Presley—one of the world's best-known music stars.

At the time of his death, Elvis Presley was forty-two years old. His reign as the King of Pop Music

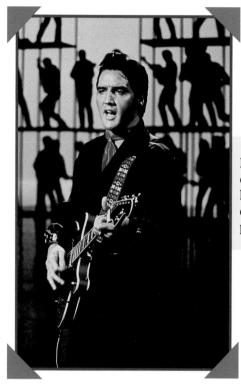

Elvis Presley's continual use of amphetamines to energize his frequently weary and overworked body was made public after his death.

could have easily continued for many more years. His fame and music lives on, but his life came to a sudden end while he was still in his prime. Presley's continual use of amphetamines to energize his frequently weary and overworked body was made public after his death. The use of amphetamines to "perk" him up along with the use of barbiturates to calm him down was a deadly factor in the King's untimely demise.[1]

The Show Biz Life

In the world of entertainment, there is an old saying, "The show must go on!" Many performers, including Elvis Presley, come to rely on the "quick fix" stimulant powers of amphetamines. These drugs include

Dexedrine™ (commonly known as little golden hearts), Biphetamine™ (commonly known as black beauties), and other chemically created substances that stimulate the central nervous system and combat fatigue.

Fans expect performers to deliver high-intensity shows no matter how the stars really feel. Amphetamines provide short-term, instant energy but they are not a safe substitute for real rest and relaxation. Stimulants, which are sometimes called speed, uppers, or bennies, are highly addictive and extremely dangerous.

Country Music Hall of Fame and Rock and Roll Hall of Fame member Johnny Cash talked openly about the lure of amphetamines.[2] Cash became dependent on Dexedrine and many other stimulants in the early stages of his career. He used uppers and alcohol to keep going and going until he absolutely had to rest. Then he used barbiturates (downers) to sleep.

The upper and downer roller-coaster ride for Johnny Cash contributed to the failure of his first marriage and his overall health. At one point, the six-foot two-inch singer was so thin that he weighed only 150 pounds.

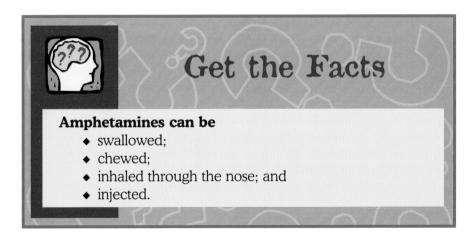

Get the Facts

Amphetamines can be
- swallowed;
- chewed;
- inhaled through the nose; and
- injected.

Once, he collapsed during a meal with food still in his mouth.[3]

Johnny Cash got help—before it was too late. Personal determination, the aid of caring friends, and professional assistance helped Cash beat his dependency.

Amphetamines and Other Occupations

No one knows for certain when or how Elvis Presley was first introduced to the addictive world of amphetamines. As a young man, Elvis worked as a truck driver before he was discovered as a singer.[4] Truckers who spend long hours behind the wheel have been known to use amphetamines. The pills hold off exhaustion and the need to sleep during lengthy trips.

Soldiers and military personnel have quietly long relied on amphetamines to remain alert during moments of crisis in prolonged combat or during boring, extensive tours of guard duty. Private (and later Sergeant) Elvis Presley may have discovered "pep pills" during his tour of duty in the United States Army.[5]

Get the Facts

Copilots is an old slang name for amphetamines. The name comes from the fact that some truck drivers on long trips use amphetamines to stay awake rather than using a relief driver to take over the driving when they become exhausted.

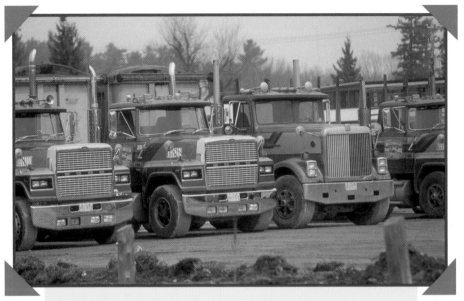

Truck drivers who spend many hours behind the wheel have been known to use amphetamines. The pills help drivers avoid feeling sleepy behind the wheel.

Curbing the Appetite

Some amphetamines are also used as diet pills. Amphetamines increase metabolism—the process by which our bodies create energy—and are believed to reduce appetite. Elvis Presley constantly watched his weight. Did he use amphetamines to control his appetite? No one knows for certain. All that is known for sure is that Presley did have an amphetamine and barbiturate problem that he battled for most of his life.

Elvis Presley also battled constant insomnia (inability to sleep) and often went whole nights at a time without any sleep at all. He may have unwisely used speed to jump-start himself after restless nights. Pep pills were known to be part of Presley's life on the road.[6]

Get the Facts

Drug abuse refers to the use of drugs or chemicals in any way that is not medically approved or which is not considered socially acceptable in a particular culture.

Later in Elvis Presley's career he was known to use large doses of powerful stimulants to energize his sleep-deprived and exhausted body. They helped to meet the demands of performing two live shows every night. Elvis Presley never disappointed his fans, but the eventual cost to his health, both mental and physical, was extremely high. At the time of his death from heart failure, an exam revealed that his body contained fourteen different drugs.

Elvis Presley died at his home, Graceland, in Memphis, Tennessee, not on tour or on a movie set. The constant cycle of using amphetamines to "pep up" and barbiturates to "calm down" becomes a trap. It is a cycle that cannot be easily broken. Presley was known to be a habitual user of Dexedrine and Biphetamine in the later years of his life.

The King Is Dead

The king of rock and roll is gone. He left behind a legacy of music and films. His drug difficulties, however, should be a lesson to others, especially those abusing amphetamines and barbiturates. Unfortunately, entertainers still turn to and abuse drugs such as amphetamines. All too frequently newspapers print the names of celebrities who admit to stimulant abuse and seek help in ending their addiction to uppers.

Others at Risk

Individuals in show business are not the only ones who risk stimulant addiction. Amphetamines are still a deceptively attractive alternative to sleep for truck drivers and students cramming for tests and exams.

Dieters hoping to curb their need for food may seek out amphetamines as may ordinary people suffering from depression. Athletes who believe they can heighten their

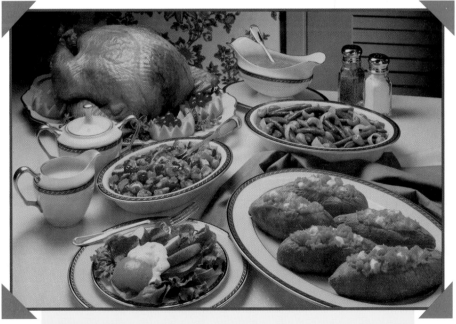

Some people will use amphetamines as a means to lose weight or curb their appetite. However, amphetamines only lead to more problems than overeating.

performance level in competitions risk possible addiction in exchange for the momentary thrill of the win.

There is no doubt that the lethal lure of amphetamines appeals to a wide range of potential abusers. Many years ago amphetamines were thought to be a type of superman drug—giving people the power to do things beyond normal human strength and endurance. Uninformed people still think of amphetamines that way—a serious and dangerous mistake.

The truth is, amphetamines are not a super cure-all for exhaustion, overeating, depression or other ailments. They are highly addictive drugs that can have a deadly effect on those who abuse them. Some see stimulants as a way to live life in the fast lane. It has been said before, but it is worth repeating . . . speed kills. There is an important lesson to be learned from the troubled life of Elvis Presley. Amphetamine abuse is dangerous and can also be deadly.

two

The Deadly Down Side of Uppers

According to research done by the Drug Abuse Warning Network (DAWN), quarterly emergency room episodes due to amphetamine use were significantly up in 1997–98 after slight decreases at the end of 1995 and the beginning of 1996. Nationally, amphetamine use and the problems generated by its abuse have continued to climb.

Perhaps one explanation for these alarming statistics is the fact that some people do not view the nonmedical use of amphetamines as a danger.

"Sure, I frequently use uppers when I cram for mid-terms and finals," a student at a major eastern university admitted. "They're easy to get and they help me stay alert and focused when I'd rather be nodding off. No, I don't have a prescription for them, but what's the harm? It's not like I'm smoking crack or using heroin. I'm not hurting anyone and I'm certainly not putting anyone in danger."[1]

It is obvious that the student who made that claim did not understand the dangerous implications of his actions. In addition to the potential harm to his own health, he broke the law by illegally using a dangerous, restricted substance. In his own small way, he participated in criminal drug trafficking.

Many people, like that student, are unaware of the consequences of stimulant abuse. This uninformed group maintains a casual acceptance of the increased overuse of amphetamines in modern society.

A survey of emergency room reports of amphetamine overdoses in select major cities around the United States supports an increase in the abuse of uppers.[2]

Easy to Get

Amphetamines are easy to obtain, which contributes to the abuse problem. Stimulants are created by people in laboratories and usually are made legally. Unfortunately,

Get the Facts

Street names for amphetamines include speed, bennies, pep pills, dexies, black beauties, hearts, jollies, uppers, bumblebees, and footballs.

Stimulants include drugs such as Dexedrine™, Biphetamine™, Ritalin™, Preludin™, Methedrine™, Desoxyn™, Tenuate™, Lonamin™, and Tepanil™.

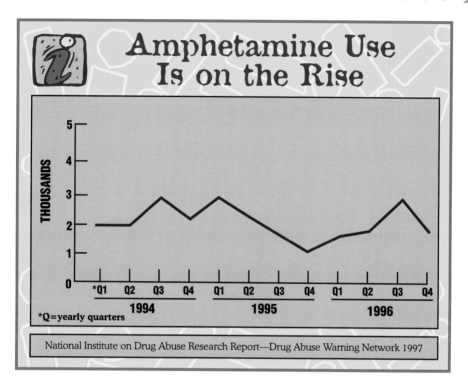

Amphetamine Use Is on the Rise

National Institute on Drug Abuse Research Report—Drug Abuse Warning Network 1997

they are often illegally distributed through various forms of criminal activity.

The easy accessibility of amphetamines to drug dealers makes them attractive and profitable. The increase in illegal amphetamine traffic raises the crime rate.

It's a Crime

In England, a twenty-eight year old single mom suffered from overwork and depression. She found that holding down a job and caring for her five small children required more energy than she had. She turned to her doctor for help.[3]

The woman's doctor wrote her a prescription for

Drinamyl™, an amphetamine combined with a barbiturate commonly called purple hearts. The Drinamyl helped the young parent feel revitalized, but she eventually developed a dependency on the drug. It got to the point where she could not get through the day without using large doses of Drinamyl. Her children and her job put great demands on her time. There were not enough hours in the day to meet the hectic requirements of her busy schedule and to get the sleep she desperately needed. Her tolerance for the drug increased, and she needed more and more Drinamyl. Tolerance is defined by the National Institute of Drug Abuse (NIDA) as a condition in which higher doses of a drug are needed to produce the same effect or high originally experienced by

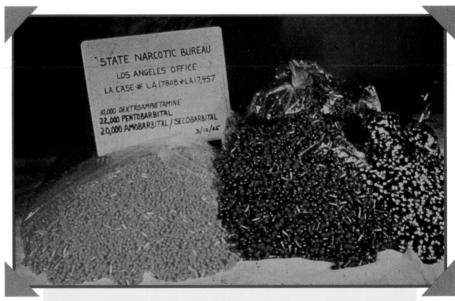

Amphetamines are often made and sold illegally. The piles of pills shown here were confiscated by the Los Angeles, California, office of the State Narcotics Bureau.

Get the Facts

A nonheart shaped form of Drinamyl (a mixture of amphetamines with barbiturates) is known by the street name "french blue."

Amphetamines produce feelings of alertness and euphoria. The ability to stay alert enables the user to go without sleep for relatively long periods.

the user. Increased tolerance often leads to physical dependency.

When the young mom's doctor suspected a developing problem, he cut back on the woman's prescription. When she had trouble obtaining a legal source for the drug, the young mother turned to criminal means to satisfy her craving. She began to illegally write her own prescriptions. Eventually the woman was caught and arrested.

The woman's use of Drinamyl proved to be a problem rather than a solution. She was sent to a rehab center for drug abuse. Her children were taken away from her and put in temporary foster care. Instead of helping her cope, the drug she relied on for relief destroyed the things most important to her.

Abuse and Its Dangers

Amphetamines are addictive both physically and psychologically. A physical addiction occurs when a person's body actually needs the drug to function. A psychological addiction is the firm belief that the drug is necessary when in reality it is not. Taking amphetamines affects not only how the body works, but also how a person thinks and sees the world.

As in the case of the young mother hooked on Drinamyl, users slowly build up a tolerance to amphetamines. The tolerance develops gradually as the need for dosage increases as much as a hundred fold.

Signs and Symptoms

The physical signs of large doses of amphetamines are recognizable. Abusers may experience dizziness, headaches, and blurred vision. They may look pale and feel hot. Their mouth may be dry and they may sweat excessively. After taking a large dose of stimulants, the abuser can suffer a loss of coordination and be affected by tremors that cause the body to shake. Often an abuser can suffer a complete physical collapse.

The way abusers see and respond to the world under the influence of amphetamines is also noticeable. People affected by stimulants may act paranoid, or unrealistically suspicious of everyone. They can be extremely self-conscious of their behavior. Amphetamine users can demonstrate compulsive behavior and talk excessively. Their actions may become repetitive. Abusers may be less organized or experience severe mood swings without reason. The simple actions of others are frequently misinterpreted. Users may think everyone is against them. Abusers can demonstrate antisocial behavior or become overly aggressive and combative. They may start fights over nothing. Stimulant users may see things and hear things that do not exist.

Amphetamines can cause severe anxiety, paranoia, and a distorted sense of reality, making those who abuse them a dangerous threat to society and to themselves.

Lost in a Sea of Stimulants

A young English woman regularly taking Dexedrine for fatigue and weight reduction suddenly disappeared from her home. For almost a week she remained missing while her parents frantically searched for her. The missing woman wandered for five days. The woman believed she was being tested and saw "special" signs that prompted her to leave home. Luckily, she finally turned up at a relative's home. She was in a state of confusion and disarray, but unharmed.[4] The Dexedrine brought on delusions which provoked her disappearance.

The Big Crash

Users of amphetamines who drive on our roads and highways put themselves and others at risk. Stimulants keep weary operators of motor vehicles awake and

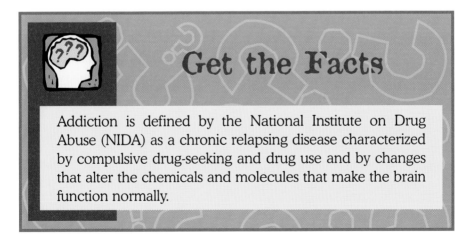

Get the Facts

Addiction is defined by the National Institute on Drug Abuse (NIDA) as a chronic relapsing disease characterized by compulsive drug-seeking and drug use and by changes that alter the chemicals and molecules that make the brain function normally.

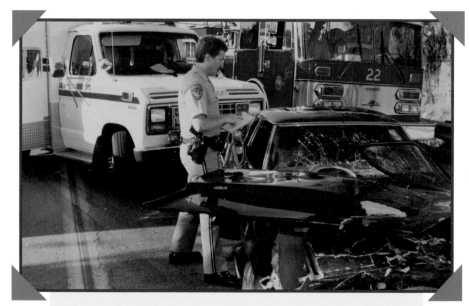

Users of amphetamines who drive on our roads and highways put themselves and other drivers at risk. While amphetamines may put off the need for sleep, they do not provide the rest that the body and mind need in order to function.

seemingly alert, but often at a terrible cost. Remaining awake does not provide the rest needed by a tired mind and body. It puts off the need to physically sleep and to mentally relax. It is like purchasing something with a credit card. You can put off paying the price for the moment, but sooner or later the bill will be due.

Amphetamines stimulate an exhausted person. They fool the body and mind into feeling energized. However, the temporary feelings of energy, alertness, and cheerfulness eventually wear off. It is then that the user may pay a steep price.

When the effects of the stimulant fade, the user can come crashing down to reality. Physical and mental exhaustion are greatly intensified due to the burning up of stored energy reserves. Abusers have been known to drop into deep sleep that lasts from twenty-four to forty-eight hours.[5] Drivers coming down from amphetamine highs have collapsed behind the wheel while their cars or trucks were still moving. Out-of-control vehicles have veered across medians and off roadways, causing serious and sometimes fatal accidents. Innocent people have died.

People who use amphetamines while driving cars and trucks pose a deadly threat to themselves and to others on the road. The use of alcohol with stimulants greatly impairs a driver's ability to operate a vehicle and intensifies the danger. It also contributes to an increased accident rate.

Risky Weight Loss

Doctors know amphetamines have a high potential for abuse. They prescribe amphetamines for use in appetite control only in cases where other types of therapy for obesity have failed. Even when amphetamines are used by physicians to help overweight patients, they are dispensed sparingly. Amphetamines are used only on a

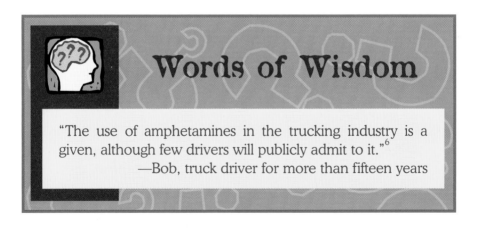

Words of Wisdom

"The use of amphetamines in the trucking industry is a given, although few drivers will publicly admit to it."[6]
—Bob, truck driver for more than fifteen years

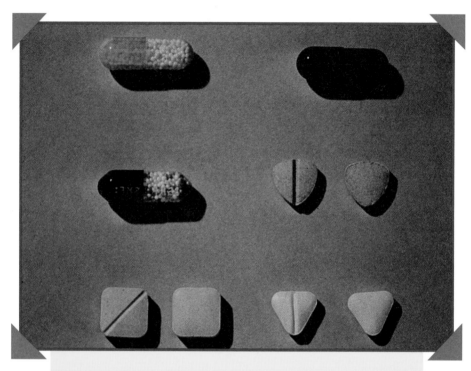

Doctors may prescribe amphetamines like the ones shown here in cases where other types of therapy for obesity have failed.

short-term basis (a few weeks). The problem with so-called diet pills is the temptation for long-term abuse.

Many years ago amphetamine dependence may have started when the drugs were prescribed by a doctor for weight loss and then abused. Today, most abuse can be traced to illegal distribution of amphetamines. However, diet pill addiction and dependency is still a serious concern.

Heavy users of diet pills often lose all interest in food and sometimes can become weak from hunger. Continued use of these amphetamines can result in a severe dependence and deterioration of the user's health.

People trying to lose weight may end up jeopardizing their health in cases of amphetamine abuse.

Even when it becomes apparent that a user's health is suffering, the continued craving for diet pills is difficult to ignore or deny. Users sometimes start to sell amphetamines and thus become criminally involved in drug distribution. The compulsive effects of physical and psychological dependency can make users violent and dangerous. The amphetamine trap snares many kinds of unsuspecting victims. The use of diet pills has to be carefully supervised.

Athletes Lose With Amphetamines

Some athletes, willing to win at any cost, take a serious risk with the nonmedical use of amphetamines. They know stimulants can enhance their performances for short periods. Take the case of a sprinter in the 100-yard dash. The difference between finishing first or second in a race may be a few tenths of a second. Because amphetamines briefly improve performance, a runner, hoping to gain an edge over competitors, might be tempted to experiment with their use.

However, the short-term gain of temporary success is overshadowed by the physical dangers to even the most superbly conditioned athlete. Amphetamines greatly increase blood pressure and heart rate. Even healthy young athletes have suffered fatal heart attacks from the use of amphetamines before, during, or after athletic competitions. Increases in blood pressure can also cause the rupture of blood vessels in the brain, producing strokes (an episode during which the brain is deprived of blood and life-giving oxygen). A stroke causes part of the brain to die and most often results in some type of

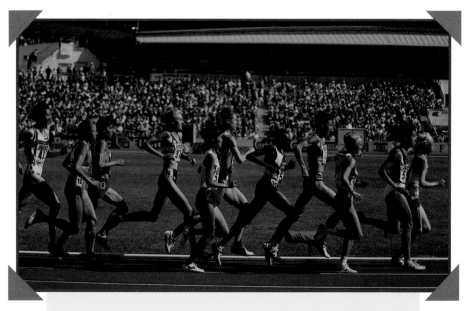

Because amphetamine use can briefly improve the performance of a runner who is hoping to gain an edge over his or her competitors, some athletes might be tempted to experiment with the drug.

paralysis, or sometimes death. Is winning a race or scoring a touchdown worth a person's life?

Officials in charge of amateur and professional sports do not support a win-at-all-cost attitude. The use of performance-enhancing stimulants is not only frowned upon, but also illegal and banned. The phrase "natural athlete" means natural. There is nothing natural about amphetamine use to boost performance. All over the world, sports organizations at every level are coming together to ban the use of drugs in athletic competitions. Athletes who use drugs are banned from future athletic events.[7]

In 1998, the International Olympic Committee (IOC) held a meeting in Lausanne, Switzerland, to discuss concerns about the use of performance-enhancing drugs among Olympic athletes. The IOC has a long list of banned drugs their athletes must avoid in order to compete. It also has a no-tolerance policy when it comes to drug use. Potential Olympic hopefuls must steer completely clear of amphetamines and other drugs if they ever hope to realize their dreams of competing for medals.

Other sports organizations also enforce tough drug restrictions. In 1998, two top United States cyclists were suspended from competing in the world's greatest bicycle race, the Tour de France, due to the use of performance-enhancing drugs. The National Basketball Association (NBA), the National Football League (NFL), the National Hockey League (NHL), Major League Baseball (MLB), the National Collegiate Athletic Association (NCAA) and other sports organizations all have tough drug-testing procedures and requirements designed to weed out abusers.

Get the Facts

Footballs is slang for amphetamine sulfate capsules. The name comes from the stimulant's oval or football-like shape.

Nigerian basketball center Julius Nwosu was suspended from playing for two months when he tested positive for a banned stimulant substance at the 1998 World Basketball Championships.[8]

Fumbled Chance

Once a college football quarterback desperately wanted to play professional football. After a tryout with an NFL squad, he was let go. He then signed with a highly competitive semipro team, hoping to improve his skills for a season in anticipation of another NFL tryout the following year. As a member of a semipro team, the ex-college quarterback had to hold down a regular day job in addition to practicing with his semipro squad in the evenings. Semipro players do not earn enough to pay all their living expenses, so they need another job. Secretly, he resorted to the use of amphetamines to "pep up" his performance at practice.

At first, his newfound energy gave him a slight edge over his competition. Gradually, however, over the season, the use of stimulants affected his weight, attitude, and concentration. His moody behavior alienated his teammates. He often lost his temper, making him unpopular. He began to believe that his offensive linemen purposely refused to block for him. Eventually, the former top athlete was demoted to second and then to third string. Finally, he was cut from the team. Amphetamine use had quickly ended his playing career. He never made it back to the National Football League.[9]

Strong-Willed Athletes

Police captain Jeff Greczyn, chairman of the County Narcotics Commanders' Association of New Jersey, discussed the problem of amphetamine abuse in a 1999 interview. "The people who are the strongest in this world are the people who never get involved with drug use and who never get addicted," he explained.[10]

Get the Facts

Amphetamines are stimulants. Stimulants increase the activity of chemicals in the part of the brain that controls our ability to pay attention and to stay alert.

Legitimate Uses for Amphetamines

Recent surveys reveal that approximately 2 percent of school-age children in the United States are currently being treated with stimulant medications for Attention Deficit Hyperactivity Disorder (ADHD).[11]

The most common stimulant used by physicians to treat ADHD is Ritalin™, a mild central nervous system stimulant. In normally functioning individuals Ritalin stimulates activity. However, in ADHD cases, it has the opposite effect. Ritalin actually helps the ADHD brain to focus better, increasing concentration and cutting down on distractions. Ritalin has a calming effect on hyperactive children and a focusing effect on children with AHDH. Exactly how it works is not understood. However, it is an integral part of a total treatment program for ADHD. It is used to help individuals affected by moderate to severe distractibility, short attention span, impulsive behavior, hyperactivity, and emotional instability.

The positive effects of Ritalin include a decrease in hyperactivity and behavior problems. Children using the stimulant also demonstrate a tendency for improved

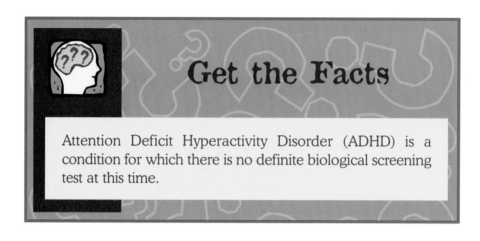

Get the Facts

Attention Deficit Hyperactivity Disorder (ADHD) is a condition for which there is no definite biological screening test at this time.

learning. However, careful and cautious professional supervision of the drug is required.

Dangers

No stimulant, including Ritalin, is free of danger or of dependency. Ritalin poses a threat to patients with a history of drug dependence or alcoholism. Such patients may try to increase Ritalin dosage on their own. Abuse can lead to marked tolerance and psychological dependence.

Other Adverse Reactions

Patients who have problems with anxiety, nervous tension, or agitated behavior—a more physically aggressive type of hyperactivity—may also react adversely or negatively to Ritalin.

The most common adverse reactions to Ritalin are nervousness and insomnia (difficulty sleeping). Children may also suffer loss of appetite, weight loss, and abdominal pain. These problems are usually solved by a decrease in dosage.

New Treatments

The value of Ritalin use in cases of youngsters diagnosed with ADHD is still the subject of debate. Ritalin has been proven effective but it is a stimulant, which in itself can be a cause for concern. In 1999, research by small independent groups working with children affected with ADHD made public claims that non-drug therapies could also be equally successful in most cases. Further study is currently going on. The future results of that research will undoubtedly affect the lives of thousands of American children currently using Ritalin.

Disturbing Reports

A 1998 survey of teenagers, teachers, and principals by the National Center on Addiction and Substance Abuse at Columbia University in New York provided some disturbing drug insights.[12]

More than half of middle school students, including

Get the Facts

Ritalin is often called "West Coast" by stimulant abusers. It is sometimes mixed with heroin, cocaine, or both for a more potent effect.

Illegal forms of Ritalin appear to be more readily available in Texas and Michigan than anywhere else in the country. Michigan historically has one of the highest per capita levels of distribution.[13]

sixth graders, reported that drugs were used, kept, and sold at their schools.

Even more alarming, three fourths of high school students said drugs were sold, kept, or used at their schools.

These beliefs may not be factual. However, they show that young people feel an ominous drug presence in their places of learning. And *learning* is the key word. The more we learn about the dangers of drugs such as amphetamines, the better our chance of avoiding the pitfalls of abuse and dependency.

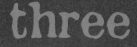

On the Alert

According to a 1998 national survey that polled American youth, the most important problem facing twelve- to seventeen-year-olds was drugs.[1] Violence, sex, and peer pressure did not come close to drugs as the top concern of American youth for the fourth straight year.

In the same survey, teachers, principals, and students concluded schools would be drug free only when the teachers, principals, and especially the students *wanted* them to be drug free.

Being drug free sounds like an easy task, but it is not. The attraction of drugs is not easy for some to resist.[2] Take Tanya (not her real name). She was not a member of the elite, popular crowd in middle school. She did not have fancy clothes or a lot of money to spend. And she was not considered pretty by her peers. Tanya was shunned and teased by her classmates. Going to

Get the Facts

The United States federal government spends $17.1 billion a year to fight drug abuse while illegal drug lords make an estimated $52 billion a year on drug sales.[3]

school was pure torture for her. Tanya did not feel very good about herself. To escape the pain she felt, Tanya turned to the one friend who welcomed her with open arms—the local drug dealer.

At the age of fourteen, Tanya began a downhill drug journey that lasted almost fifteen years. During her drug abuse, she used speed, LSD, cocaine, and other drugs. In high school she barely weighed one hundred pounds and saw her career hopes of participating in dance and gymnastics vanish in a drug-induced haze. After high school during a weekend binge, she suffered a seizure and a heart attack that almost killed her.

Shortly after her close call with death, Tanya, then in her midtwenties, decided to break the drug chains that held her prisoner. Personal determination, newfound religious convictions, and the help of friends, loved ones, and professionals led Tanya back onto a drug-free path.

The long journey ended on a happy note for this former drug user, but for many others who choose the same road, the trail leads to disaster. Life is a series of important choices we all have to make. Not all people make the right choices.[4] One addict under arrest in

Maryland shouted to the judge he stood before, "I hustle. I steal. I cheat. And I shoot dope. I use it because I like it."

What Would You Do?

Amphetamines, speed, and diet pills are no substitutes for studying in advance, being mentally and physically ready to play a sport, maintaining a proper diet, and being comfortable with your appearance. The temptation to use drugs can appear in many ways and forms. It is not always easy to resist a quick-fix solution to a problem.

Stay Alert

A friend plans to take amphetamines to stay up all night to cram for an exam on the following morning. She invites others to do the same because a good grade will help a grade-point average. What should she know?

Make the Right Call

A starter on the middle school basketball team about to play for the league championship sees a teammate use amphetamines in the locker room before the game

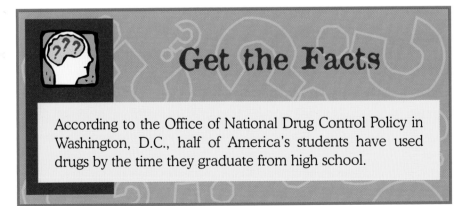

Get the Facts

According to the Office of National Drug Control Policy in Washington, D.C., half of America's students have used drugs by the time they graduate from high school.

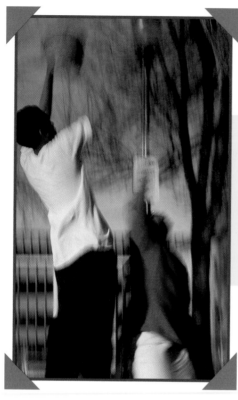

Amphetamines might seem like a tempting choice to the star basketball player looking for an edge on the court. But, the long-term problems associated with the use of amphetamines do not justify the momentary glory.

begins. The amphetamine user is a star player. What should the other player do?

Weigh the Consequences

The biggest school dance of the year is only weeks away and a friend would like to lose a few pounds, but there is not enough time to diet properly. She attempts to lose the weight by taking some of her mother's prescription diet pills. What should she know?

There are some telltale signs of amphetamine use that can help in detecting possible abuse. The following questions may indicate a friend or relative's need for help. If the answer is yes to a majority of the following questions, amphetamine use is a real possibility.[5] If a friend might be abusing stimulants and needs help to overcome a dependency, he or she should talk to an adult who can help.

1. Does this person go long periods without sleep or feeling tired?

2. Does this person have an unexplainable loss of appetite or a strange revulsion for eating?

3. Does this person have odd, moody spells, becoming short-tempered and hostile?

4. Does this person sweat a great deal, suffer spells of dizziness, or have dilated pupils in the eyes?

5. Does this person believe everyone is out to get him or her, even though there is no evidence of that?

6. Does this person have a lot of clumsy, little accidents and not seem to be paying attention?

7. Does this person chatter on and on, constantly repeating words, phrases, or stories?

8. Does this person nod off and sleep soundly for a long time (twenty-four to forty-eight hours) after long periods of extreme activity?

9. Does this person confess to hearing and seeing things others do not?

10. Does this person get angry with others for no real reason?

In 1999, the Office of National Drug Control Policy in Washington, D.C., began a five-year, $2 billion antidrug ad campaign aimed at young people aged nine to nineteen.[6]

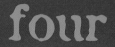

four

The History and Effects of Stimulants

Stimulant use and possibly abuse probably dates back hundreds of years.

The native people of Latin America were chewing the leaves of a plant to produce a stimulant effect long before the arrival of the first Spanish explorers in the fifteenth century. Those were coca leaves from which the drug cocaine is derived.

Amphetamines, artificially made stimulants, were first produced in 1887. The drug Benzedrine was first used medically in 1935 as a treatment for narcolepsy (a sleep disorder). The first nonmedical use of Benzedrine occurred during the Spanish Civil War in 1936. Amphetamines were included in the survival packs of some soldiers involved in the conflict.

The German Army began to issue amphetamines to its soldiers in 1936. Stimulants were viewed as a helpful energizer for soldiers suffering from stress and fatigue. The German high command saw no problem (mentally or physically) with the use of amphetamines and regularly distributed stimulants to soldiers for routine use.

When World War II arrived (1939–1945), amphetamines were being widely used by both sides especially in combat. In fact, some 72 million amphetamine tablets were issued to British soldiers alone during the conflict. The stimulants kept troops on the alert at times when they would normally be too exhausted to focus or continue.

After the war, the nonmedical use of amphetamines gradually appeared in the workforce and in the home.

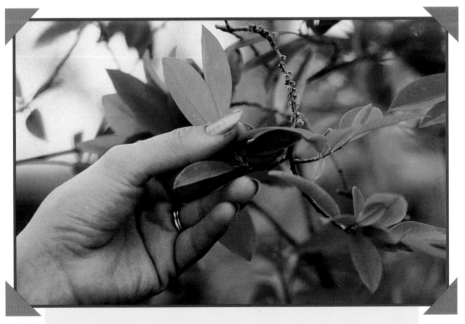

Use of stimulants dates back hundreds of years. The native people of Latin America were chewing coca leaves to produce a stimulant effect long before the fifteenth century.

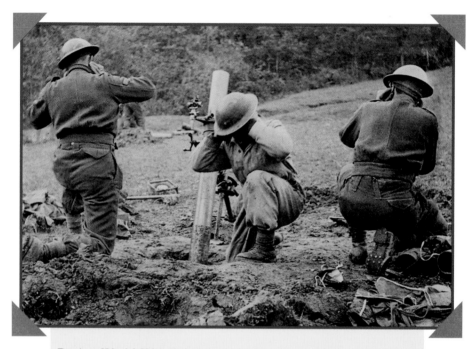

During World War II (1939–1945) amphetamines were widely used by both sides, especially in combat situations.

Research done by England's D.R. Davis in 1947 found amphetamines could help people perform tasks faster, even when exhaustion set in. People did not, however, perform better with amphetamines than if well rested.[1]

People in professions where fatigue was a factor, such as truck drivers, entertainers, and night watchmen, came to rely on the energizing effects of amphetamines. Depressed, overworked, and sometimes slightly overweight housewives of the period were also prime targets for amphetamine abuse.

In the 1950s and 1960s, teenage abuse of amphetamines began to surface. Prescription pills were often taken from unsuspecting parents for illegal use.

In the 1970s, at the peak of the Vietnam War, there

was an interest in many types of drugs. Once again, amphetamines seemed an attractive method of squeezing more wakeful hours into exhausting, hectic schedules.

In the 1980s and 1990s, the busy pace continued. A growing interest in sports made athletes keenly aware of the enhanced performance possibilities with various stimulants and amphetamines.

How Amphetamines Get Into the Body

Usually amphetamines are prepared so an initial dose is released immediately, and the remaining dosage of the medication is gradually released over a longer period. Sustained time-release amphetamine products should never be crushed or chewed by the user because this increases the effects. However, abusers often do just that.

Amphetamines also come as short-acting pills, such as Ritalin, used primarily for children with ADHD. With short-acting pills, one dose of medication is required in the morning, and one is needed in the afternoon.[2]

Get the Facts

The three prime medical reasons for the prescribing of amphetamines today are
1. narcolepsy (sleep disorder);
2. Attention Deficit Hyperactivity Disorder (ADHD); and
3. excessive weight gain (obesity).

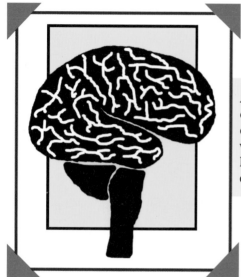

Amphetamines affect brain chemistry by causing some chemicals to be released when they should not be. Because of this, brain activity does not slow when it should.

The Action of Amphetamines

Amphetamines cause increased blood pressure. They also have a weak stimulating effect on breathing. The most pronounced effect of amphetamines is on the brain where they affect brain chemistry. They trick the brain into disregarding some information while feeding it other conflicting information. Simply put, amphetamines cause brain chemicals to be released when they should not be. Brain activity does not slow down even when it should.

Excessive Weight Gain (Obesity)

Stimulant drugs used to treat obesity are known as diet pills. It has not been proven that they suppress appetite, even though most people believe that they do. Some researchers believe the pills may fool or trick the brain into believing the stomach is already full and the blood has sufficient fuel.

The amount of weight lost with diet pills varies from

case to case. The rate of weight loss, however, is always greatest in the first two weeks of therapy. Diet pills are recommended only as a short-term solution for losing weight and should be combined with an exercise and nutrition plan. Tolerance does develop and can be dangerous. Patients become tempted to exceed the recommended dose in an attempt to increase weight loss. At that point the drug should not be increased but discontinued.

Another health problem associated with diet pills is malnutrition. The user frequently does not get enough minerals and vitamins because he or she is just not hungry. When a person does stop using amphetamines to stimulate weight loss, food cravings quickly return. The user experiences a strong feeling of hunger that is

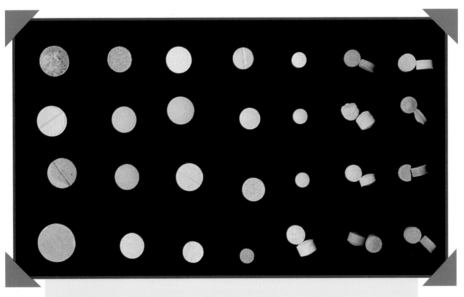

While amphetamines can be used for weight lose, they should be used only as a short-term solution and should always be combined with an exercise and nutrition plan.

Words of Wisdom

"If you want to fight the war on drugs, sit down at your own kitchen table and talk to your children."[3]
—United States Department of Education

sometimes even greater than the person's original appetite.

The Amphetamine Abuser

Abusers of amphetamines can develop deep depression, delusions, hallucinations, panic attacks, and a disturbed mental state much like schizophrenia.[4] (The abuser may have attention defects, strange disturbances in behavior and activity, and odd personality changes such as thinking he or she is someone else.)

Other effects already touched on include violent and aggressive behavior, tolerance to the drug, and dependence. Physically the abuser can suffer from malnutrition, blockage of blood vessels, infections resulting from injections, and increased susceptibility to illness (due to poor diet, lack of sleep, and generally bad health).

Amphetamine Overdose

Individuals will respond differently to amphetamine overdose. The usual symptoms are restlessness, tremors, rapid respiration, mental confusion, combative aggression, hallucinations, and panic attacks where a person paces back and forth.

Physically, an overdose can cause an irregular heartbeat, vastly increased blood pressure, and circulatory collapse. Other problems include nausea, vomiting, diarrhea, and stomach cramps. Fatal overdose cases are usually preceded by convulsions and coma. Death may also occur due to burst blood vessels in the brain, heart attacks, or very high fever.

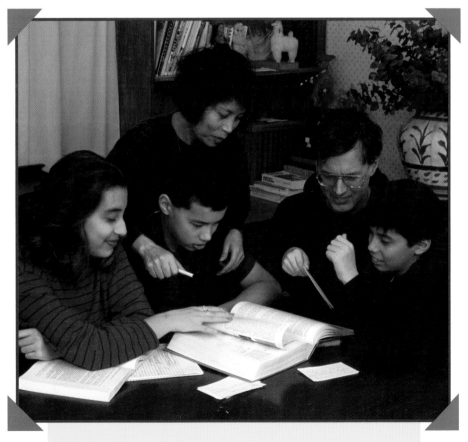

Parents who want to "wage the war against drugs" need to sit down and talk to their children.

Withdrawal

When amphetamine use is suddenly halted, symptoms just the opposite of the drug's usual effects occur. The user becomes extremely tired or sleepy, a condition that may last for several days. Sleep is long but disturbed. In addition, the individual may experience such deep and severe depression that suicide is a possibility. There may also be delusions and hallucinations. Extreme hunger and severe exhaustion are also present. Reassurance by comforting friends or loved ones and a quiet, peaceful environment help a person recover. Withdrawal should always be closely supervised by a physician. In some cases prescription drugs may be used to ease the withdrawal symptoms.

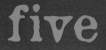

The Battle Against Abuse

All across the United States and Canada, more schools may soon require their students to pass a drug test to participate in extracurricular activities—from athletics to the Honor Society. The practice of testing all students (not just athletes) who want to participate in activities such as Drama Club, Yearbook, and the Math Club is slowly gaining acceptance.[1]

Testing Programs

In Rush County High School in Indiana, drug testing of all students involved in extracurricular activities has been going on since 1996.

Some schools in Florida, Idaho, Pennsylvania, and California have followed suit. Educators are sending a clear message to their students: If you want to be involved in school activities, steer clear of drug use.

Prevention

The best way to combat drug abuse is to be aware of its dangers and to actively get involved in the battle against drugs. The first and most important step is not to use stimulants. The next step is to help others avoid the traps of drug abuse.

Be Aware

There is no such thing as being too young to know about drug dangers. Experts on drug abuse state that by the third grade, a young person should know what an illegal drug is, why it is illegal, what it looks like, and what harm it can do. They should also know why it is important to avoid unknown and possibly dangerous substances. Students even in elementary schools should know not to share stimulant medications such as Ritalin with their classmates and friends.[3]

Get Involved

Peer group programs have proven to be a successful way for friends to help friends combat drugs. Peer helpers

Get the Facts

In 1998 the largest national youth antidrug media campaign ever undertaken by the federal government was launched. It included twenty-nine television commercials airing nationwide. The five-year campaign is estimated to cost $195 million.[2]

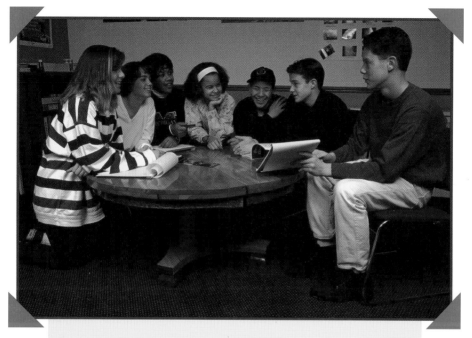

Peer helpers are teens who can talk to other teens. Peer helpers assist others in making wise life choices—such as resisting the temptation to do drugs.

assist others in helping themselves make wise life choices. Peer helpers are sometimes called peer counselors, peer buddies, or peer tutors. Instead of adults preaching the dangers of drug use, peer helpers provide continuous student-to-student dialogues. There are no judgments and no pressure to do the "right" thing. One prime concern of peer helpers is how to refuse the temptation of drugs. Peer helpers can also be a bridge between troubled students and adult professionals.

Peer helpers have to undergo some training. It is not difficult or boring. It is a fun way to help students at the same age level or younger. Youth organizations, church groups, and schools can all sponsor peer help programs.

Words of Wisdom

"I did drugs for fourteen years. For me [staying clean] is an everyday event for the rest of my life."[4]

—Tanya, recovering addict

Listen and Learn

Drug Abuse Resistance Education (DARE) is one drug prevention program brought to schools by law enforcement workers. It is usually aimed at fifth or sixth graders. Rather than centering on the harmful effects of particular drugs such as stimulants, it attempts to help students recognize the pressure that may influence them to experiment with any drugs.

Another type of drug prevention program takes a hard-line approach. Former drug addicts and recovering drug abusers under police supervision deliver antidrug speeches to youngsters. The programs usually are presented with local and state police antidrug organizations. The presentations are truthful, poignant, and sometimes scary. They provide young people with the harsh realities of real drug abuse. The ex-addicts talk about their chilling, real-life experiences on the street.

Athletic Coaches Get Involved

Unfortunately, some athletes turn to performance-enhancing stimulants. In the United States and Canada, high school coaches are taking steps to ensure their athletes remain drug free. In schools that do not have mandatory drug-testing policies, many coaches are requiring members of their sports teams and the parents of athletes to sign drug-free pledges at the start of the season. Coaches are also taking part in drug-awareness programs, to recognize the symptoms of stimulant or other drug use by their players. In addition, coaches are becoming more active in mentoring roles off the athletic field. They hold regular team meetings that stress honest communication, positive peer pressure, and training rule enforcement. Their goal is to create a safe place for confidential coach-athlete conferences. Many coaches are now using drug survey sheets, like the following example, to poll their athletes on drug usage.[5]

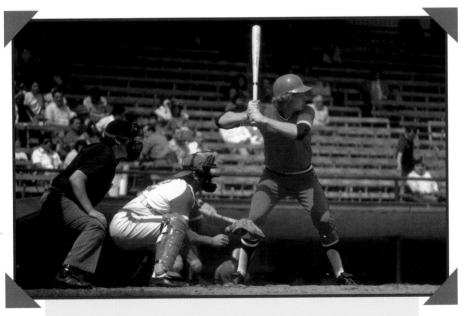

Many schools and coaches are taking more active roles in keeping their athletes drug free.

Sample Confidential Coach's Survey of Drug and Alcohol Use Among Athletes

The purpose of this survey is to gather information about the use of drugs and alcohol among student athletes. Please be honest about your experiences and feelings. All responses are strictly confidential. DO NOT PUT YOUR NAME ON THIS PAPER. Circle the appropriate answer or answers.

1. Male   Female

2. Grade: 6th 7th 8th 9th 10th 11th 12th

3. Did you use any of the following substances during the last sports season?

       Amphetamines (speed, uppers) Y / N

Crack Y / N	Downers Y / N
Alcohol Y / N	Cocaine Y / N
Marijuana Y / N	LSD Y / N
Steroids Y / N	Tobacco Y / N

       Other Drugs Y / N

4. Did you use any of the above substances during the last month? Y / N

5. Which, if any? _____

6. Would you go to a party where alcohol or other drugs are being used? Y / N

7. Have you ever felt that you have a problem with alcohol or drugs? Y / N

8. Do you know someone on your sports team who has an alcohol or drug problem? Y /N

9. Does a member of your immediate family have a problem with alcohol or other drugs? Y / N

10. How can we as teammates (coaches and players) stop drug use by our athletes?

Programs to Help Drug Abusers

There are many different types of drug rehabilitation programs. Some are more effective than others. The bottom line between success and failure seems to depend a great deal on the individual drug abuser. The key is to find the right program for each person.

Innovative drug treatment programs around the country, such as Freedom House in New Jersey, are finding ways to help abusers break their drug chains. Freedom House is a very successful, no-nonsense, residential program for recovering substance abusers. The program is designed to put structure back into the shattered lives of substance abusers. Its goal is to effect a change in behavior.[6]

The patterning seems to work. Statistics show that 87 percent of Freedom House graduates since 1985 have remained drug free.

Structured Environment

A typical day of rehab at highly structured substance abuse centers such as Freedom House starts before dawn for its residents. They shower, eat breakfast, and fix a bag lunch. Then it's off to work. All residents are required to have outside jobs, which are overseen by their house staff. Residents are taken to work and later picked up. Back at the center, dinner is followed by chores and various group meetings. Residents' schedules are tightly packed. In all, a resident living at a place like Freedom House may get only an hour of nonstructured free time per day.

Incoming clients at residential treatment centers are faced with rigid rules. At Freedom House there are no phone calls, letters, or newspapers available for the first two weeks. Appropriate behavior by new residents brings privilege rewards and more free time. After months of appropriate behavior, residents can earn weekend passes. Staff members continually rate residents' performances and check with employers to evaluate on-the-job output and attitude.

There is not much individual freedom for the residents of places like Freedom House. The freedom comes from being drug free. Recovering substance abusers are subject to unannounced room checks and random searches. Any infringement of house rules or problems on the job result in immediate and severe cutbacks of privileges. The program may sound harsh, but it is working where some less strict treatment programs have failed.

six

Fighting

Back

It takes real courage to refuse drugs. Young people often see others their own age or older abusing substances such as amphetamines. That substance abuser may be a relative, family member (parent or sibling), or a close friend. It may be someone who is respected, admired, or considered just plain cool. That is often the case with amphetamine and stimulant abuse.[1]

Deciding not to do drugs is not so easy when others send the messages that it is okay to break the law.

Refusal

It may be a bit easier to refuse drugs after considering questions such as the following: Does true happiness come from drug use or rather from good, strong relationships with other people? Is the time spent with loved ones and those who care about you better than the time spent doing drugs? Would it be better to use the money spent on drugs for legitimate forms of relaxation and entertainment such as live concerts or movies?

No superman

Amphetamines were once considered "superman" drugs. There are no real supermen or wonderwomen. Everyone gets tired. Many people have dealt with some type of weight problem at one time or another. All athletes lose sometimes. There is nothing wrong with being human. People must find productive ways to cope with problems, setbacks, and failures.

Even the Best Fail

Michael Jordan, one of the greatest basketball players of all time, tried to play professional baseball and discovered he could not hit well enough to advance to the major leagues. He was disappointed, but he dealt with it. He did not use drugs; he went back to playing basketball.

The point is, there is always an alternative to substance abuse. Drugs, whether they be stimulants, amphetamines, or other illegal substances, are not part of the solution. They only compound the problem. No matter what others say or do, taking a pill is not how winners cope.

Avoiding Temptations

If a person is in a group where someone uses speed or other drugs, how easy will it be to refuse the use of a controlled substance? It will be very difficult. It will require a great deal of willpower, true courage, and high moral values.

Sometimes, the best way not to fall into a trap is to avoid the path that leads to it. Do not just blindly follow your friends to parties or other social gatherings. Ask questions like these:

- Is this party a place to have good, clean fun?
- What kind of kids will be at this party?
- Will there be any adults around in case there is trouble?[2]

If a friend wants to go to a place where drugs are available, suggest an alternative. Take charge.

It may not be easy, but try to hang out with friends who do not need drugs or alcohol to socialize and have fun. Friends who need drugs to enjoy themselves are not friends worth having.

Refusing Drugs

Morgan (not his real name) joined a drama group and turned his back on his so-called musician buddies when

Words of Wisdom

"Today's pulse check shows that the work of America's parents, teachers, and public officials is far from done. America's young people need to have a single, unambiguous message—drugs are wrong and dangerous, and they can kill you!"[3]

—President Bill Clinton

they suggested he try drugs. Morgan later starred in several community plays and even wrote a play that was produced at the local community college. He got his highs taking bows in front of appreciative audiences.

Saying no works best when it is combined with another action—leaving. There is no standard answer that works every time for refusing to try speed, amphetamines, or other drugs. Everyone, young and old, has to look deep inside to find the good sense and willpower to refuse. We have to be strong together as families, as communities, and as a nation to solve our drug problems.

questions for discussion

1. Are the nonmedical uses of amphetamines safe?

2. A classmate hands you a pill before an exam and says it will help you concentrate better. What do you do?

3. A star athlete on a sports team uses performance-enhancing stimulants. Is it fair to his teammates? Should you tell someone?

4. Truck drivers sometimes claim amphetamines help them do their jobs better. Do you agree?

5. Is there anything wrong with using someone else's diet pills to lose a few pounds?

6. What do you think about the fact that entertainers often use nonprescription uppers to put on a good show for their fans?

7. How difficult or easy does becoming addicted to amphetamines seem to be?

8. Why were amphetamines once thought to be a superman drug?

9. What are the signs of amphetamine overdose?

10. Why do you think amphetamine use is on the rise?

11. Why are some people more likely than others to try amphetamines or other stimulants?

chapter notes

Chapter 1. Life in the Fast Lane

1. Albert Goldman, *Elvis* (New York: Avon Books, 1981), pp. 413, 414.

2. VH1 Music Network, "Legends Documentary—Johnny Cash," February 7, 1999.

3. Ibid.

4. W. A. Harbinson, *The Illustrated Elvis* (New York: Tempo Star, 1977), p. 16.

5. Goldman, pp. 347–356.

6. Ibid.

Chapter 2. The Deadly Down Side of Uppers

1. Author interview with Rutgers University student J. H. (September 1998).

2. National Institute on Drug Abuse Research Report, Drug Abuse Warning Network 1997.

3. Peter Laurie, *Drugs, Medical, Psychological and Social Facts* (New York: Penguin Books, 1969), p. 81.

4. P. H. Connell, *Amphetamine Psychosis* (Englewood Cliffs, N.J.: Prentice Hall, 1958), p. 23.

5. Narcotic Educational Foundation of America, Amphetamine Abuse (Rockville, Md.: Narcotic Educational Foundation of America, 1991), p. 1.

6. Author interview with professional truck driver R. S. (September 1998).

7. "Drug Abuse," News Brief, *The Sunday Courier News*, (Bridgewater, N.J.), August 2, 1998, p. B1.

8. Stephen Wilson, "IOC Focuses on Drugs," *The Courier News* (Bridgewater, N.J.), August 20, 1998, p. C4.

9. M. J. Pellowski, "Recollections of Semipro Football in the 1970s," unpublished article, Hartford, Conn., 1971–72.

10. Michelle Sahn, "Ex-User Hopes Story Scares Kids Straight," *The Courier News* (Bridgewater, N.J.), September 28, 1998, p. A1.

11. Jeffrey Kirchner, "Long-Term Amphetamine Use in Children with ADHD," *American Family Physician*, April 1998, p. 67.

12. National Institute on Drug Abuse, General Drug Information, "Ritalin," p. 20.

13. Joseph Califano, Jr., "Talking About Drugs" *The Courier News* (Bridgewater, N.J.) November 1, 1998, p. A 14.

Chapter 3. On the Alert

1. Michelle Sahn, "Ex-User Hopes Story Scares Kids Straight," *The Courier News* (Bridgewater, N.J.), September 28, 1998, p. A4.

2. Robert Guy Matthews, "Free From Heroin's Grip— Minister Tends to Others," *The Baltimore Sun*, April 7, 1998, p. A7.

3. Joseph A. Califano, Jr., "Talking About Drugs," *The Courier News* (Bridgewater, N.J.), November 1, 1998, p. A14.

4. "War Against Drugs Turns to Classrooms, Homes," *The Sunday Courier News* (Bridgewater, N.J.), January 17, 1999, p. A6.

5. Mark A. de Bernardo, *Guide to Dangerous Drugs* (Washington, D.C.: Institute for a Drug Free Workplace, 1995), pp. 10–11.

6. Rex W. Huppke, "Drug Smugglers—Cops Matching Wits on Interstates," *The Sunday Courier News* (Bridgewater, N.J.), January 17, 1999, p. A6.

Chapter 4. The History and Effects of Stimulants

1. D.R. Davis, *Psychotic Effects on Analeptics & Their Relation to Fatigue Pneumonia in Air Crew* (New York: Wiley Publishing Co., 1964), p. 145.

2. National Institute on Drug Abuse, General Drug Information, "Ritalin," p. 20.

3. "War Against Drugs Turns to Classrooms, Homes" *The Sunday Courier News* (Bridgewater, N.J.), January 17, 1999, p. A6.

4. United States Department of Education, *A Parent's Guide to Prevention—Growing up Drug Free* (Washington, D.C.: U.S. Department of Education, 1998), p. 34.

Chapter 5. The Battle Against Abuse

1. Steve Rhodes, "Drug Test the Chess Club," *U.S.A. Weekend*, November 20, 1998, p. 14.

2. Michelle Sahn, "New Commercials Try to Unsell Kids on Drugs," *The Courier News* (Bridgewater, N.J.), September 28, 1998, p. A6.

3. Barbara B. Varenhorst, *Real Friends* (Becoming the Friend You'd Like to Have) (New York: Harper & Row, 1983), p. 182.

4. Michelle Sahn, "Ex-User Hopes Story Scares Kids Straight," *Courier News* (Bridgewater, N.J.), September 28, 1998, pp. A1, A4.

5. United States Department of Justice, Team up—A Drug Prevention Manual for H.S. Athletic Coaches (Washington, D.C.: U.S. Department of Justice, Drug Enforcement Administration, 1998, pp. 6, 9, 10, 11.

6. Mark Terenzi, "Golfing for Freedom," *The Courier News* (Bridgewater, N.J.) July 16, 1998), pp. 1, 3.

Chapter 6. Fighting Back

1. United States Department of Health, *Keeping Youth Drug Free* (Washington, D.C.: U.S. Department of Health and Human Services, Substance Abuse and Mental Health Services Administration, 1998), p. 7.

2. United States Department of Education, *Growing up Drug Free, A Parent's Guide to Prevention* (Washington, D.C.: U.S. Department of Education, 1998), p. 8.

3. Gail Repsher, "Methamphetamine Use Skyrockets," *The Courier News* (Bridgewater, N.J.), October 12, 1998, p. 8.

where to write

American Council for Drug Education (ACDE)
204 Monroe Street
Rockville, MD 20852
301-294-0600

Drug and Alcohol Abuse Prevention and Treatment
Department of Justice, Room 758
633 Indiana Avenue NW
Washington, DC 20531
202-724-8491

Institute for a Drug Free Workplace
1225 O Street NW
Suite 2000
Washington, DC 20005
202-842-7400

National Clearinghouse for Alcohol & Drug Information (NCADI)
P.O. Box 2345
Rockville, MD 20852
1-800-729-6686

National Families in Action
2957 Clairmont Road, Suite 150
Atlanta, GA 30329
404-248-9676

National Peer Helpers Association
P.O. Box 335
Mountain View, CA 94042
415-965-4011

The National Network for Youth
1319 F Street NW
Suite 401
Washington, DC 20004
202-783-7949

Internet Addresses

Community Anti-Drug Coalitions of America
< http://www.cadca.com >

National Clearinghouse for Alcohol Abuse & Drug Information (NCADI)
< http://www.health.org >

National Families in Action
< http://www.emory.edu/NFIA/ >

National Institute on Drug Abuse (NIDA)
< http://www.nida.nih.gov >

Office of Minority Health Resource Center
< http://www.onmrc.gov >

Youth Power
< http://www.youthpower.org >

further reading

Berger, Gilda. *Drug Abuse*. New York: Franklin Watts, 1998.

Chomet, Julian. *Speed and Amphetamines*. New York: Franklin Watts, 1990.

Clayton, Lawrence. *Amphetamines and Other Stimulants*. New York: The Rosen Publishing Group, Inc., 1994.

Jaffe, Steve L., ed. *Amphetamines and Other Uppers*. New York: Chelsea House Publishers, 1999.

Kuhn, Cynthia. *Buzzed: The Straight Facts About the Most Used and Abused Drugs From Alcohol to Ecstasy*. New York: W. W. Norton & Company, Inc., 1998.

Lukas, Scott E. *Amphetamines: Danger in the Fast Lane*. New York: Chelsea House Publishers, 1992.

index